Little known facts about infectious diseases

Imaging on crossroads

Constantin Panow

Copyright 2016

All rights reserved

Printed by Createspace

"About medications that are drunk or applied to wounds it is worth learning from everyone; for people do not discover these by reasoning but by chance, and experts not more than laymen."

Hippocrates (460-370BC)

Disclaimer

The author and publisher decline responsibility about any wrong interpretation or misunderstanding and flawed application of principles exposed in this short text.

Copyright 2016	1
Disclaimer	2
Purpose of title	5
Publish or perish!	6
Toll of Earth	7
Why me	7
Examples	9
Silhouette sign revisited	9
Mycoplasma pneumonia	9
Clinical diagnosis	10
Labs	10
Cold agglutinins!	10
Radiology	11
Description	11
OA	12
Justification	14
Viruses!	15
Differential	17
Aspergillus	18
Parasites	19
Nematodes	19
Ascaris	19
Eelworm	20
Pinworm	21
Flatworms (Platyhelminthes)	23
Importance of ultrasound	24
Special cases	25
Arthritis	26
Neuritis	26
Alternative to serology	27

Splenomegaly	28
Kidney	29
Pyelonephritis	29
Pyelitis	30
Full-blown	31
Doppler imaging	31
Normal Kidney Doppler	31
The case of prostate gland	32
Focal prostatitis	32
Total gland involvement	32
Virus	32
Punctiforme pattern	33
Chronic prostatitis	34
Liver	34
Acute hepatitis	34
Normal liver size	35
Granulomatous hepatitis	36
Other granulomas	36
Chronic hepatitis	36
Steatosis characteristics	37
Spleen anatomy	37
Multiplicity of disease	38
Genetics	39
Website	39

Purpose of title

Evidence based medicine has been a thorn in the eye (or in the ass) of many practitioners.

If a lot has been published, and is well known, nowadays it becomes more and more difficult to satisfy the public;

Not to mention the higher realm of University.

Every diagnosis is supposed to be proven twice, but if possible by some kind of extra-terrestrial force, rather than by our intelligence alone!

Even measles in children who have not been vaccinated must sustain demonstration through serology.

No more clinics!

We, old clinicians, have to be happy that our descendants and nowadays Professors of Medicine have not invented a method to prove measles through biopsy.

Even more thankful, that they do not request a

probe of brain tissue examination under microscope!

Publish or perish!

On the other hand « Publish or perish! » has made more difficult for our *species* to withstand the glorious advance of Medicine in University.

So-called *Reviewers* refuse systematically publications of some of us to permit to other ones to bring the very same material a few months later in their paper, almost unchanged.

Copyright applies to a fulfilled task as a publisher, and not to ideas as such!

Thus, the idea, true scaffold of any work, and which is promoting any article or book becomes in reality trustworthy good of any owner who would put it in print.

Toll of Earth

The only fact, which nowadays professors forget in this Eden Garden, is that Medicine is equal to hard work.

If you want to earn a jewel, you must descend far down underground, where those blossoms are resplendent in the light of Darkness.

The whispering realm that voices never share,
« No one dares! »

In this way many a pearl have been collected by some individual on the edge of suffocation, like the treasure of genetics for which it is said that a depressive assistant worked for years, and two other ones earned the necklace.

Why me

So, to make a long story short, I decided to publish a small text of little known, but already (for most of them) published facts in Modern Medicine;

For which you can research all by yourself to find proof in outstanding texts, which other medical workers have written.

Not precisely for myself!

But, who knows, if I am not their testament grand-son?

As medicine has been for myself more than a profession, but rather a passion and a lifelong quest for knowledge;

I decided to recollect for you this short story from old books and journals.

If you are like me, you would enjoy it!

(Well, I hope so...)

If not, you would rather say, or write: « Really?! »

Let's start with

Examples

Silhouette sign revisited

First one:

Mycoplasma pneumonia

This is most common lung inflammation during the "bad season".

Sometimes you can tell that patients are coming from opposite hemisphere on Earth during summer.

In warm season occasional cases are to be observed in people who bath for longer time, and thus cool down their bodies for protracted periods.

Summer disease has also typical and different picture on chest X-Ray from winter illness, as infiltration is more confluent;

That is, we call it acinar, or streaky, and hilar and mediastinal lymph node enlargement can be present and is thus conspicuous.

Clinical diagnosis

How do you diagnose this common disease during predilection season?

Well, the patient comes to you complaining of cough with little white sputum.

In 10-15% of cases he/she has chest pain.

(As involvement is, as you would see on further description, peripheral, pleural and sub-pleural! And concerning dependent areas of lung.)

Labs

D-Dimeres can be extremely elevated.

CRP and white cell count can be high or normal.

Patient remembers further spontaneously, or on directed questioning having « *numb hands* »at night.

Cold agglutinins!

As you can order them for a lab proof of this

disease.

Or, it is sufficient to put a sample of blood in your fridge, or outside your window in winter.

Radiology

But, most of the time, practitioners would ask first for a chest X-Ray.

Of course, everyone knows that such interstitial infiltrates of atypical pneumonia can be diagnosed on *high resolution* CT. (*Ground glass appearance*). *High cost* indeed!

But, reviewing my old knowledge of thorax radiology I rediscovered (about 10-15 years ago) with this entity the « *silhouette sign* »,

(Described 1950 by Drs Benjamin and Henry Felson).

Description

Mycoplasma pneumonia is responsible for

disappearance of contour of right hemi-diaphragm (40%);

Left hemi-diaphragm (30%);

Or right heart border (35%);

Exceptionally left heart limit (<5%).

Most frequently involved structure is *medio-basal* or *para-cardiac segment* of right lower lobe, involved in more than 55% of cases.

Right and left hemi-diaphragm are concerned together in 35% of pneumonias approximately. Right hemi-diaphragm and right atrial limit in 30-35%.

In this way, chest X-Ray is a very efficient modality to solve clinical problems.

OA

Osteo-articular system and Mycoplasma pneumonias

It occasions inflammatory process at tendinous insertions, not unlike other bacteria, similar to any

Fiessinger-Leroy-Reiter disease.

If we start with this end of a spectrum, you can envision all infectious diseases under the aspect of their accompanying osteo-articular participation.

It is very interesting to notify that each germ attacks a specific point or structure.

Thus, as I mentioned already, insertionitis belongs to bacteria

(And Mycoplasmas, to be mentioned separately as they are obligatory intra-cellular pathogens!).

On the long run this produces, for instance, calcaneal spurs, or vertebral beaks.

They also attack not seldom articulations with true arthritis, to be differentiated from septic arthritis only by its importance, which is heaviness of bacterial burden inside synovia.

Remember the so-called « *facet syndrome* », a typical manifestation of Reiter's syndrome.

Apart from insertions of tendons on bone, they can cause also typical teno-synovitis, with one word, every part of the body where we find synovia.

Or, bursae!

Again, calcaneal spurs...

Bursitis!

Justification

Why do I find my expose useful in nowadays medicine?

Because we can see those fine structures with imaging modalities and differentiate between them!

Progressing further on spectrum of germs, we find other obligatory intra-cellular bacteria, which are Chlamydia and alike.

Typically they are supposed to be part of STDs, but I think they only secondarily migrate to gonads, but are primarily air-transmitted disease.

They are said to remain asymptomatic in testicles (Low-grade epididymitis) and ovaries (Slight PID) and only occasionally flare-up as a peri-hepatitis (Fitz-Hugh-Curtis syndrome in females).

OA

In musculo-skelettal tract they provoke a pathognomonic picture in Achilles tendon with thickening of this structure and slight peri-tendinitis.

Observe!

No inflammation at insertions, bursae, or articulations (As far, as I know!)

Last, but not least, we arrive at the end of this short list:

Viruses!

Everybody knows what a flue is!
Strong muscle pain.

OA

Myalgia, which can be focal or diffuse, here we

can further pinpoint agent of aggression.

Some cause a true myositis, which you can see on MRI with special methods (Injected with fat sat).

One half of scapular girdle (right or left involvement) is typical for *Parvo-virus*.

Inter-costal myalgia or myositis is classic for Coxsackie and Echo-viruses.

For Flu diffuse muscle pain is typical.

(Almost indistinguishable from post-exercise catarrh).

Labs

Muscle enzymes can be elevated.

Cardiac involvement is also frequent: *Myocarditis*!

OA

Further, viruses attack cartilage.

They provoke typically so-called *Tietze syndrome*. You can observe it with ultrasound as a slight effusion along rib-cartilage.

If there is no fissure underneath, you know viral disease is at hand.

Differential

Some viruses, like Parvo-virus are so aggressive, that they imitate a true arthritis with liquid in articulations.

Now you understand also why some patients present with bronchitis, and why there is further evolution towards bronchi-ectasia in protracted disease in childhood, or with whooping cough. (Respiratory syncitial virus for instance, responsible for bronchiolitis in small children).

Bordetella pertussis is supposed to be a bacterial agent, but its symptoms are resistant to antibiotics. (Not the germ itself!)

Disease could be a combination between a bacterium and virus.

Aspergillus

Mushrooms, yeast and alike have tropism for different structures, but are rare diseases.

The most common, Aspergillus, and also one of most aggressive ones tackles apart from ciliated epithelium of broncho-pulmonary system, smooth muscle and provokes thus so-called *allergic aspergillosis*, which is almost equivalent to asthma.

Apart from the fact, that involvement is more on the side of bigger bronchi, than bronchioles.

Further, plugging in those structures produces bronchi-ectasia.

OA

Consecutive bacterial superinfection is responsible for osteo-articular complaints.

Parasites

On the side of parasites, tropism is manifold, depending on type of germ.

OA

Unicellular ones, like *toxoplasmosis*, are seen more frequently in muscle tissue, but can involve any structure, including eye (Chorio-retinitis).

Nematodes

Ascaris

Intestinal parasites, if true ones, like Ascaris (*Ascaris lumbricoides*) are prompt to travel through bowel wall and other structures, like bile ducts and liver, searching a way of reproduction with mates.

Size in freshly infested human bowel is 1mm (0.039inches) in transverse diameter and 5cm in length (1.97inches).

Worm measurement is one reliable tool for

diagnosis.

OA

Traveling outside abdomen is rather rare for this kind of parasite, but transgressing intestinal wall can cause all sorts of septic pictures.

Eelworm

Strongyloides stercoralis, Eelworms and other Nematodes are readily visible with modern high resolution ultrasound probes in intestinal lumen.

Strongyloides stercoralis has a size of about 0.2-0.4mm (0.0079-0.016 inches) in transverse section with a length of about 2-4mm (0.079-0.16 inches). *Measurement with ultrasound permits its diagnosis in bowel.*

This small size allows the worm to travel through vessel walls, and to provoke a true sepsis with negative hemo-cultures!

OA

Hence, all human anatomy is exposed to it, but most frequently radiologists diagnose it in lungs (Loeffler's syndrome).

Pinworm

Pinworm, or *Enterobius vermicularis* is still said in modern Textbooks on Parasitology to be a parasite. In fact, it is rather a saprophyte, present in every human on Earth, and essential for our well-being and immune system and proper digestion of meals. It rarely produces disease;

Sometimes a slight pain and itching in right iliac fossa in spring;

Or when the sun has eruptions and more electromagnetic activity.

Then it is high time for them to mate, most often in spring or autumn. (North Hemisphere, Europe)

Some years of high sun activity they are particularly prone to proliferate, and this for several years in human bowel.

Second syndrome seen in women is urethritis, and sometimes you can pinpoint them with ultrasound in the bladder of this gender.

Size is 0.8mm (0.031 inches) in transverse diameter, and 8 mm in length (0.31inches).

Old females can attain 5 cm length (2 inches).

In this second situation they are especially numerous in sigmoid colon, where you can elicit slight sensitivity or pain on pressure with your ultrasound probe, and old females are in big proportion, but also hence you can see longer worms, able to travel outside anus.

OA

In sigmoid colon females erode sometimes mucosa, and permit transgression of bowel wall by bacteria.

Thus I observe frequently facet syndromes in this situation.

So much for round worms (Nematodes).

Flatworms (Platyhelminthes)

Most feared of their representatives are Taenias (Tapeworms).

Cysticercosis of brain is an ominous picture, hence importance of an early diagnosis.

Those worms have become extremely uncommon in industrialized society, and I can recollect only one case in my personal experience with ultrasonography.

This modality is best suited for early diagnosis, but difficulty resides in the fact that the worm is flat, and in one direction transverse diameter would not exceed 0.8mm (0.031inches).

Following the structure along bowel wall over several cm (several times 0.4inches) would provide you with the right diagnosis.

Recognizing that the worm is flat, and its second

diameter on transverse section is much bigger is another challenge, same as observing at first glance that bowel wall is *"double"* in some sections on the inner part, and over a short distance...

OA

Cysticerca ca travel through all human anatomy, but are more readily observed in muscle. (Calcified granulomas)

Importance of ultrasound

As long as we do not dispose of PCR (plasma chain reaction) test for diagnosis in parasitology, or analogue test, measuring worms in human bowel is a reliable alternative for diagnosis.

Laboratory medicine brings confusion to this topic.

We know now that pinworm eggs are seen on stool specimens only exceptionally, thus the scotch tape test, which is said to be more reliable.

Special cases

One bacterium outside the spectrum of usual ones is Borreliosis (*Borrelia burgdorferi*).

Europe and North America are endemic for this disease, as far as ticks have their predilection area. Here, again, early recognition can be useful.

If, in most cases, healing is almost instantaneous, and it is this way for populations exposed since centuries and thousands of years to this disease, other genetic constitution of humans, originating from non-endemic areas could be an issue.

Neuro-borreliosis, with meningitis and encephalitis is one serious situation.

Culture would be negative.

Thus, diagnosis relies on serology, PCR and other clinical signs and symptoms.

Less acute presentation of illness consists of two typical syndromes.

Arthritis

First one is *arthritis*.

Its differential on clinical grounds is difficult, but not so on radiological ones.

Inflammation is obvious, with synovia proliferation, effusion in joint, hyper-vascularity of synovia on Doppler, strong enhancing on MRI.

But, even days after initiating event you don't observe any bone destruction or erosion **at all**. Tendon insertions are spared with this germ.

Thus, if you have symptoms along extremity, search for complication number two, which is *neuritis*.

Neuritis

Peripheral nerve thickening is readily seen with high resolution Ultrasound probe, and there are *"jumping nodes"*.

They can attain several times the size of concerned nerve, but most of the time do not exceed twice normal diameter.

This disease is most common cause for neuritis in endemic areas.

Serology is reliable only to 50%.

Thus, if you are not sure about disease, and want a further proof, toss a coin!

You would spare some money.

Alternative to serology

But, if patient consults the first week after beginning of symptoms, you have still another option for establishing definite diagnosis.

Germ is extremely sensitive to tetracycline.

Do following test: Prescribe Vibramycine! (A tetracycline antibiotic).

In the case of Borrelia-induced arthritis the patient is asymptomatic within 3 days, and in the case of neuritis within one week.

Splenomegaly

The case of slight splenomegaly

Though this entity is reported in literature with impressive lists of diseases, and thus differential diagnoses (DDs), to which it is supposed to be companion;

I see it in regular clinics mainly (almost only?) in 3 common conditions:

. Most frequently with Epstein-Barr disease (infectious mononucleosis), for which you can have a hint if the patient presents with pharyngitis (Most of the time starting a few days before examination).

. Chlamydial disease (The patient complaints of dysuria, prostatitis, or salpingitis, pelvic inflammatory disease, PID).

. Vibrio infection (Vibrio haemolyticus and para-haemolyticus which goes with under-cooked or uncooked sea-food consumption a few hours earlier!)

Kidney

The case of kidney infection

Most commonly occurs in women.

This is not a sign of persisting vesico-ureteral reflux, affects most commonly normal anatomy.

Pyelonephritis

Most of the time presentation is best visible on ultrasound, as *focal pyelonephritis*.

It concerns upper pole of kidney in females sleeping on their back, and lower pole in those, less frequent situation, who spend most of the night on the tummy. (10-15%)

The explanation of this fact is, of course, because of orientation of this organ in the sagittal plane. Dependent portions have a bigger chance to be involved.

Image shows hyper-echogenic triangle with apex

around a calix.

Or, rather a pyramid pointing toward a unit of two or three such *"glasses"*.

Not to be confused with an already present scar from a previous infection, as both show a lot of *whitish material* on ultrasound, because of fat and collagen in scar tissue.

Pyelitis

Second, less common presentation is *pyelitis*, where you have no parenchyma participation, or almost.

In this situation prominent sign is thickening of walls of pyelon and caliceal system.

This sign can attain 2mm (0.079inches), but most of the time is less obvious, in vicinity of 1.5mm (0.059inches) rather.

In my practice I see less than one pyelitis for 10 focal pyelonephritis cases.

Full-blown

Kidney disease

Exceptionally, you would see total kidney participation, which is fortunately very seldom, and occurs only in long lasting untreated urine infection.

Neglected by patients themselves!

Doppler imaging

On Doppler, triangle of focal inflammation presents with hypo-perfusion in the middle, which means lower velocities, but higher RI;

While surrounding area is distinguished by hyper-perfusion, which is accelerated blood flow in arcuate arteries, with lowering of resistances (RI).

Normal Kidney Doppler

Normal velocities in inter-lobular renal arteries are 25-35 cm/sec (9.8-13.8inches/sec), and RI navigates usually in vicinity of 0.55-0.65.

The case of prostate gland

Focal prostatitis

Here again, focal inflammation is most common presentation in bacterial disease.

Concerned area is strongly hyper-echogenic.

Unfortunately Doppler is not contributive in my experience.

Total gland involvement

Exception to this rule is Chlamydial infection, where distribution of inflammation is more even, and concerns most of the time the whole gland. (But, less hyper-echogenic than first picture.)

Virus

Completely regular, but less "whitish" pattern is

diagnostic for viral disease.

Punctiforme pattern

Vesical gland (vesiculae seminales) disease can be diagnosed on ultrasound if there is a small dot-like hyper-echogenic focus at mouth of those "bags" in prostatic urethra.

As those structures are able of contraction; Inflammation, though bacterial, is most of the time clinically silent.

Bleeding, though, frequently occurs, with tinged ejaculate accordingly.

MRI shows blood degradation products in seminal vesicle.

As you can observe from previous expose, there is strong relationship first between echogenicity, or strength of "whitish pattern", and extent of disease on the other hand, towards intensity of clinics.

Most intense would be whole gland involvement

with bacterial disease, where you see most *septic* presentations.

Chronic prostatitis

After a few weeks and months, untreated disease produces calcified foci, which you can observe more frequently in patients with reduced immunity;

As for instance in diabetes mellitus.

Liver

This organ can be afflicted by many illnesses, so I would mention only a few of them.

Acute hepatitis

Hepatitis A is an acute disease, with a lot of cytolysis, hepatic enzymes elevation being tremendous, several 100 units/liter of SGOT/SGPT

(ASAT/ALAT), sometimes 1000 units/l.

On ultrasound the organ is enlarged.

Normal liver size

I find it most easy to define one measure in sagittal plane of middle hepatic vein, where there is least variation of anatomy, as it can be considered middle point for this organ.

Here normal measurement does not exceed 12 cm in adults (4.7 inches).

Liver edge is then rounded (obtuse) in acute hepatitis, instead of being pointed or acute (as it is normally).

Echogenicity seems unchanged.

There is frequently slight effusion around gallbladder wall.

Granulomatous hepatitis

Most common is Epstein-Barr disease. Transaminases are only slightly elevated of about 70-80 units/L.

Liver size is only just above normal, usually not more than 13-14cm in length (5.12-5.51 inches). Edge of organ is rounded.

There is no effusion around gallbladder wall.

Other granulomas

In other granulomatous illnesses microscopic lesions are visible as such, as ultrasound has a spatial resolution far inferior than 0.1 mm (0.004inches);

And structures of this minute size can be readily not only visualized, but can be measured as such.

Chronic hepatitis

B and C disease is characterized by higher liver

echogenicity, readily visible by comparison with cortex of right kidney.

Steatosis characteristics

In C hepatitis there is sometimes accompanying steatosis, which is characterized by hypo-echogenic areas in gallbladder bed and in vicinity of round ligament (segment 4b).

Distinction from simple hepatic steatosis is difficult, as elevation of liver enzymes is not prominent, and can be just borderline.

Thus, imaging diagnosis relies on spleen measurement.

Spleen anatomy

Old data, which maintain 12 cm as maximal length for a normal spleen are no more tenable. (4.7inches).

Single measurement should not exceed rather 10 cm (3.9 inches).

More precise is determination of spleen volume, to be approximated in all cases.

Every evaluation above 200 ml should be considered abnormal, in confines of slight splenomegaly (6.76 US fl oz).

Multiplicity of disease

Last but not least, old speculations pretended that only one viral disease can attack at one time the human body, because of interferon, interleukin encoding and similar highly intellectual stronghold.

Now we know, such information is pure phantasy and poetry.

Not only several viruses can coexist in the same time and colonize our bodies, but they even potentiate bacterial agents;

As this is the case of gastro-duodenal ulcer disease, due to Helicobacter pylori;

But opening again under viral attack.

Genetics

Thus, on DNA ground, we are not Martians, very terrestrial indeed, but more worm than human, and more bacterial and mold even, and even further in this same logic viral.

In the same order in which Life appeared on Earth: From simple to complex.

Viruses (Several Billions years), bacteria (3.5 Billion years), Mycelia (1.5 Billion years) and only very much later multicellular beings like worms (0.3-0.5 Billion years).

Website

I hope you enjoyed this short text.

If you have questions or comments, I would be glad to discuss it all with you:

Write in my blog!

www.thenopillshealthprospect.com

www.ingramcontent.com/pod-product-compliance
Lightning Source LLC
Chambersburg PA
CBHW061232180526
45170CB00003B/1257